103 Meal and Juice Recipes to Reduce Constipation:

Facilitate Your Digestion Using Effective and Delicious Foods

By

Joe Correa CSN

COPYRIGHT

ACKNOWLEDGEMENTS

This book is dedicated to my friends and family that have had mild or serious illnesses so that you may find a solution and make the necessary changes in your life.

103 Meal and Juice Recipes to Reduce Constipation:

Facilitate Your Digestion Using Effective and Delicious Foods

By

Joe Correa CSN

CONTENTS

ABOUT THE AUTHOR

After years of Research, I honestly believe in the positive effects that proper nutrition can have over the body and mind. My knowledge and experience has helped me live healthier throughout the years and which I have shared with family and friends. The more you know about eating and drinking healthier, the sooner you will want to change your life and eating habits.

Nutrition is a key part in the process of being healthy and living longer so get started today. The first step is the most important and the most significant.

INTRODUCTION

103 Meal and Juice Recipes to Reduce Constipation: Facilitate Your Digestion Using Effective and Delicious Foods

By Joe Correa CSN

The most common symptoms for constipation are stomach cramps, being unable to empty your bowels, or extremely hard stool. This can have psychological affects that are followed by loss of appetite and anxiety.

While it may be difficult to determine the exact cause of constipation in most individuals, one of the best cures is to increase your fiber intake through natural produce such as nutrient packed fruits and vegetables. Juicing is a very easy way to consume the fiber needed to reset your digestive system. Foods that are easily digestible and consuming them daily will allow your digestive system to rest and heal itself.

These recipes are easy to make at home and bursting with flavor and nutrients your body will crave for.

Continue drinking water while you change what you eat and drink, make sure you include light physical activity, such as a daily stroll outside to get some fresh air and enjoy the relief that will come to your body and soul as you repair your digestive system with these recipes.

This book offers great meal and juice recipes to make your dining table simply irresistible. By adding enough fiber and some specific ingredients to your diet, you can reduce, and even heal constipation in a couple of days. Try all of these recipes and see the difference!

103 MEAL AND JUICE RECIPES TO REDUCE CONSTIPATION

Meals

1.   Tender Venison Stew with Prunes

Ingredients:

21oz shoulder of venison, chopped into bite-sized pieces

1 cup of sour cream

2 ½ cup of beef broth

½ tsp of freshly ground black pepper

1 tsp of salt

5 tbsp of vegetable oil

4 large onions, finely chopped

7oz prunes, sliced

2 tbsp of fresh blackberries

1 cup of red wine vinegar

½ cup of whipping cream

1 bay leaf

Preparation:

In a small bowl, combine vinegar with bay leaf and blackberries. Pour the mixture over prunes and set aside for 30 minutes.

Heat up the oil over medium-high heat. Add chopped venison and briefly cook, 5-6 minutes. Now add chopped onions and continue to cook until translucent. Season with salt and pepper and gradually add beef broth, ½ cup at a time, stirring constantly.

When the meat is half tender, add prunes and vinegar mixture. Reduce the heat to a minimum and continue to cook for 45 minutes.

Stir in whipping cream and sour cream and serve warm.

Nutritional information per serving: Kcal: 380 , Protein: 49g, Carbs: 38g, Fats: 26g

2.   Rice Omelet with Spring Onions

Ingredients:

4 tbsp of olive oil

3 whole eggs

1 cup of rice

4 large spring onions, chopped

½ tsp of freshly ground black pepper

1 tsp of salt

Preparation:

First you have to cook the rice. Use a package directions or simply combine one cup of rice with three cups of water. Bring it to a boil and give it a good stir. Reduce the heat to minimum and cook until the water evaporates. Remove from the heat and chill. Transfer to a serving platter.

Heat up the olive oil in a large saucepan, over a medium-high heat. Whisk the eggs in a bowl and season with some salt (about ¼ tsp). Pour the eggs in a skillet and fry for 2 minutes. Flip over and cook for one more minute. Remove from the heat and slice the egss into ½ inch thick strips.

Transfer to a bowl with rice. Add some more salt and pepper and give it a good stir.

Top with chopped onions and serve.

Nutritional information per serving: Kcal: 245 , Protein: 18g, Carbs: 40g, Fats: 22g

3.   Vegetable Patties

Ingredients:

7oz carrot, sliced

3.4oz cauliflower, chopped

7oz broccoli, chopped

7oz kale, chopped

1 egg

3.5oz breadcrumbs

½ cup of all-purpose flour

2 tbsp of extra virgin olive oil

1 tsp of salt

For the sauce:

½ cup of liquid yogurt

½ cup of fat-free mayonnaise

¼ cup of sugar-free tomato sauce

Preparation:

Place the chopped vegetable in a deep pot. Add enough

water to cover and one teaspoon of salt. Cook until fork tender. Remove from the heat and drain. Chill for a while and transfer to a food processor. Pulse to combine and place in a bowl.

Whisk in one egg and flour. Using your hands, shape one inch thick patties. Dip each pattie in breadcrumbs.

Heat up the olive oil in a large saucepan. Fry each patty for 3-4 minutes on each side and transfer to a serving platter.

Prepare the sauce by combine yogurt with mayonnaise and tomato sauce. Chill for a while and serve.

Nutritional information per serving: Kcal: 276 , Protein: 39g, Carbs: 41g, Fats: 30g

4.   Broccoli Orecchiette

Ingredients:

1 pack (10oz) orecchiette

1lb broccoli

3.5 turkey breast fillet, thinly sliced

1 large onion, peeled and finely chopped

7oz button mushrooms, sliced

2 garlic cloves, crushed

½ cup of cooking cream

3 tbsp of extra virgin olive oil

1 tsp of salt

½ tsp of pepper

2 tbsp of grated parmesan

Preparation:

Heat up the olive oil in a large saucepan. Add chopped onion and stir-fry until translucent. Now add turkey breasts and continue to cook for 3-4 more minutes, stirring constantly. Now add garlic and button mushrooms, and stir well. Cook until the liquid evaporates and add cooking cream, salt, pepper, and chopped broccoli. If the mixture is too thick, you can add ¼ cup of vegetable stock. Reduce the heat, cover, and simmer for five more minutes.

Use a package instructions to prepare orecchiette. Drain and combine with broccoli sauce. Serve warm.

Nutritional information per serving: Kcal: 518 , Protein: 48g, Carbs: 53g, Fats: 24g

5.   Stewed Turkey Breast with Celery Risotto

Ingredients:

1lb turkey breast meat, chopped into bite-sized pieces

7oz long grain rice

1 medium-sized onion, peeled and finely chopped

2 tbsp of melted butter

1.5oz celery root, sliced

1 tsp of nutmeg, ground

¼ cup of apple juice

A handful of fresh parsley

1 tsp of sea salt

½ tsp of freshly ground black pepper

Preparation:

Combine oil with butter in a large skillet. Heat up over medium-high heat and add onion and celery root. Stir-fry briefly, for 3-4 minutes and add turkey breast and continue to simmer adding about ¼ cup of water at a time. Now add apple juice, fresh parsley, and ground nutmeg. Give it a good stir and briefly boil. Remove from the heat.

Meanwhile, cook the rice. You can use a package direction to prepare your rice or simply place the rice in a deep pot and add four cups of water. Cook over medium heat until water has evaporated. Stir occasionally.

Combine rice with turkey breast sauce and serve warm. You can decorate with some more fresh parsley, but this optional.

Nutritional information per serving: Kcal: 413, Protein: 31g, Carbs: 39g, Fats: 20g

6.   Steamed Chineese Spinach with Ginger

Ingredients:

14oz spinach

1 tbsp of sesame seeds

1 tsp of ginger, grated

2 tbsp of freshly squeezed lime juice

¼ cup of water

2 tbsp of olive oil

1 tsp of sesame oil

½ tsp of salt

Preparation:

Wash and clean spinach leaves. Roughly chop them and set aside.

Heat up olive oil and sesame oil in a large wok pan. Add chopped spinach and cover. Cook for ten minutes, uncover and add ginger, lime juice, sesame seeds, and water. Continue to cook for five more minutes.

Remove from the heat and serve.

Nutritional information per serving: Kcal: 209 , Protein: 5g, Carbs: 19g, Fats: 14g

7.   Turkey Breast with Garlic and Broccoli

Introduction:

1lb turkey breast, sliced into one inch thick slices

1 tbsp of cayenne pepper

5 tbsp of vegetable oil

2 large carrots, sliced

1lb broccoli, sliced

2 garlic cloves, crushed

4 tbsp of extra virgin olive oil

Preparation:

Combine five tablespoons of vegetable oil with one tablespoon of cayenne pepper. Using a kitchen brush, spread the mixture over turkey breast. Set aside in the refrigerator for 30 minutes.

Meanwhile, place sliced carrot in a pot of boiling water. Add one teaspoon of salt and cook for ten minutes. Now add broccoli and continue to cook until fork tender. Remove from the heat and drain.

Heat up the olive oil in a large saucepan and add garlic, carrot and broccoli. Gently simmer for 5-6 minutes and add turkey breast. Cover and cook for 20 minutes.

Remove from the heat and serve.

Nutritional information per serving: Kcal: 175 , Protein: 29g, Carbs: 8.6g, Fats: 22g

8.   Kidney Bean Salad with Eggs

Ingredients:

1 whole egg, boiled

1 cup of lettuce, finely chopped

½ cup of green beans, cooked

½ cup kidney beans, cooked

4 cherry tomatoes, halved

1 tsp of ground chili pepper

Few black olives, sliced

3 tbsp of extra virgin olive oil

½ tsp of salt

1 tbsp of fresh lemon juice

Preparation:

First you want to boil the egg. Gently place the egg into a pot with just enough water to cover. Bring to a boil and cook for 10 minutes. You can use a kitchen timer. After 10 minutes, drain the water and place the egg under the cold water. Peel and slice

Meanwhile, combine other ingredients in a large bowl. Add the olive oil, fresh lemon juice, and salt. Toss well to combine. Top with sliced eggs and serve.

To prevent the ingredients from changing the color in leftover salad, cover tightly with a plastic wrap. Keep in the refrigerator.

Nutrition information per serving: Kcal: 191 Protein: 45g, Carbs: 50g, Fats: 19.8g

9.   Green Bean and Radish Salad with Olive Oil

Ingredients:

1lb green beans

7oz radish, sliced

5oz cherry tomatoes, halved

1 tsp of salt

Dressing:

4 tbsp of extra virgin olive oil

1 tsp of fresh mint, finely chopped

2 spring onions, chopped

2 tsp of freshly squeezed lime juice

½ tsp of salt

Preparation:

Wash and clean the beans and place in a deep pot. Pour enough water to cover and add one teaspoon of salt. Cook for 15-20 minutes. Remove from the heat and drain. Cool for a while and transfer to a serving bowl. Add halved tomatoes and sliced radish. Toss to combine.

In another bowl, combine all dressing ingredients. Drizzle over salad and serve cold.

Nutritional information per serving: Kcal: 200 , Protein: 1.1g, Carbs: 36g, Fats: 27g

10.   Asian Curry Chicken with Prunes

Ingredients:

1lb chicken fillet, boneless and skinless

2 large red bell peppers

1 small green bell pepper

1 cup of freshly squeezed orange juice

4 prunes, pitted

1 cup of chicken broth

1 tbsp of ground curry

1 tsp of salt

¼ tsp of freshly ground black pepper

4 tbsp of vegetable oil

Preparation:

Season the meat with some salt and pour over the orange juice. Add prunes and marinate for 30 minutes. Remove the meat from the marinade and slice into bite-sized pieces.

Heat up the oil in a large wok pan and add chicken breast. Stir-fry for 3-4 minutes and add chopped, bell peppers, curry, pepper, and continue to cook for 2 more minutes.

Now add the chicken broth and bring it to a boil. Reduce the heat and simmer for 30 minutes.

Serve warm.

Nutritional information per serving: Kcal: 496 , Protein: 38g, Carbs: 40.5g, Fats: 26g

11.   Arugula Salad with Parmesan

Ingredients:

10oz fresh arugula, torn

3.5oz grated parmesan cheese

Dressing:

¼ cup of extra virgin olive oil

2 tbsp of apple cider vinegar

1 tbsp of freshly squeezed orange juice

1 tsp of dijon mustard

1 tbsp of sour cream

Preparation:

Whisk together all dressing ingredients until fully combined. Chill for 30 minutes in the refrigerator.

Place arugula in a serving bowl. Add parmesan cheese and toss to combine.

Drizzle with dressing and serve cold.

This salad tastes even better when refrigerated overnight, but that is optional.

Nutritional information per serving: Kcal: 176 , Protein: 18g, Carbs: 21g, Fats: 19g

12.   Fresh Vegetable Wraps with Greek Yogurt

Ingredients:

1 pound of chicken breast, boneless and skinless

2 cups of chicken broth

1 cup of fat-free Greek yogurt

1 cup of fresh parsley, chopped

½ tsp of sea salt

¼ tsp of ground pepper

4 cups of chopped lettuce

1 cup of diced tomato

½ cup of onion, sliced

1 package of whole grain tortillas

Preparation:

Combine chicken broth and chicken meat in a sauce pan over medium heat. Cover the sauce pan and allow it to boil. Cook for another 10-15 over medium-low heat. Remove from heat and drain. Let it stand for a while.

Chop the meat into bite size pieces. Meanwhile, in a large bowl, combine Greek yogurt, chicken meat, parsley, salt and pepper. Mix gently until the chicken is well coated.

Spread this mixture over tortillas and top with lettuce, tomato and onion. Roll and serve.

Nutrition information per serving: Kcal: 167, Protein: 21.5g, Carbs: 14.5g, Fats: 5g

13.   Lentil Burgers with Garlic

Ingredients:

2 cups of lentils, pre-cooked

3 cloves of garlic, minced

½ cup of breadcrumbs

¼ cup of reduced fat parmesan cheese (freshly grated is best, but whatever you got will work)

1 egg, beaten

2 cups of water

½ cup of rice flour

salt and pepper to taste

Preparation:

1In a medium size bowl, mash lentils with folk then mix with garlic, breadcrumbs and cheese. Form into patties; set aside. Whisk egg and water in bowl; flour and salt & pepper in another bowl.

Coat each patty gently with flour mixture, dip into egg, then coat again with flour. Over medium-high heat in a large skillet, heat oil. Fry the burgers until lightly brown, about 2-3 minutes each side.

Serve on warm bread or in a pita with cilantro, yogurt, onion, tomatoes and whatever else you like – but this is optional!

Nutrition information per serving: Kcal: 195, Protein: 19.8g, Carbs: 16.1g, Fats: 6.7g

14.   Creamy Winter Chicken

Ingredients:

1 pound of boneless chicken, chopped

1 2/3 cups of chicken broth

2/4 cup of chopped onions

½ cup of brown rice

½ cup of low-fat cottage cheese

3 tbsp of fat-free Greek yogurt

¼ tsp of salt

½ tsp of basil

¼ tsp of oregano

¼ tsp of thyme, crushed

1/8 tsp of garlic powder

1/8 tsp of pepper

Preparation:

Combine the chicken and onions into a skillet and cook between medium to high heat until chicken is cooked. This should take about 20-30 minutes.

Place chicken and onions into a large bowl and then add chicken broth, uncooked brown rice, basil, salt, oregano, thyme, garlic powder, pepper and cottage cheese. Mix up until everything is thoroughly combined.

3Place the mixture into an ungreased 1½ quart casserole dish with a tight fitting lid.

Preheat oven to 350 degrees. Bake covered for about 30 minutes, or until rice is done, stirring it several times during cooking.

Uncover the casserole dish and top with Greek yogurt.

Bake uncovered for about five more minutes until yogurt is completely melted. Garnish with parsley before serving.

Nutrition information per serving: Kcal: 198, Protein: 23.5g, Carbs: 16g, Fats: 5g

15.   Sweet Potato and Mushroom Sliders

Ingredients:

1 large sweet potato

1 cup of fresh button mushrooms

1 cup of low-fat cottage cheese

3 egg whites

¾ cup of chia seeds

¾ of a cup of long grain rice

¾ of a cup of bread crumbs

1 tsp of tarragon

1 tsp of parsley

1 tsp of garlic powder

1 cup of chopped spinach

Preparation:

Pour 1 cup of water in a small saucepan. Bring it to boil and cook rice until it's slightly sticky. This should take about 10 minutes.

At the same time, cook chia seeds until soft in a separate pot. Finely chop mushrooms. Thoroughly rinse spinach.

Mix all the ingredients together in a large bowl. Put the bowl into the fridge to chill for 15 to 30 minutes. Take mixture out of the fridge and form into patties.

Make sure cooking surfaces are cleaned and greased before adding patties to prevent them from sticking. Fry each piece on a medium temperature for about 5 minutes on both side.

Nutrition information per serving: Kcal: 186, Protein: 22g, Carbs: 19g, Fats: 5.8g

16.   Sweet Pumpkin Salad With Almonds

Ingredients:

1 cup of chopped pumpkin

1 cup of arugula

3 tbsp of chopped almonds

1 tsp of dry rosemary

½ tsp of dry thyme

Olive oil

Preparation:

Preheat the oven to 350 degrees. Grease the baking sheet with some olive oil. Spread the pumpkin and sprinkle with rosemary and thyme.

Bake for about 30 minutes.

Remove from the oven and allow it to cool for a while.

Meanwhile combine other ingredients in a bowl, add pumpkin, and some more olive oil. Serve.

Nutrition information per serving: Kcal: 180, Protein: 4g, Carbs: 28g, Fats: 2.1g

17.   Hazelnut Quinoa with Cranberries

Ingredients:

1 cup of quinoa, cooked

3 tbsp of hazelnuts, roasted

½ cup of fresh parsley

1 small onion, peeled and chopped

2 garlic cloves

¼ tsp of salt

5 tbsp of olive oil

1 cup of button mushrooms, sliced

¼ cup of cranberries, dry

Preparation:

Combine the hazelnuts, parsley, salt and 3 tbsp of olive oil in a food processor.

Blend well for 30 seconds.

Heat up the remaining olive oil in a large skillet. Add chopped onion and garlic. Stir well and fry for several minutes, until nice light brown color.

Add cooked quinoa, button mushrooms, and mix well. Cook for 5 more minutes, until the water evaporates. Remove from the heat and transfer to a bowl. Add hazelnut mixture and ¼ cup of cranberries.

Mix well and serve warm.

Nutrition information per serving: Kcal: 160, Protein: 17g, Carbs: 31g, Fats: 12g

18.   Lentil Stew with Turmeric

Ingredients:

10oz lentils

tbsp of canola oil

1 medium-sized carrot, peeled and sliced

1 small potato, peeled and chopped

1 bay leaf

¼ cup of parsley, finely chopped

½ tbsp of turmeric powder

Salt to taste

Preparation:

Melt the butter in a medium-sized skillet. Add sliced carrot, chopped potato and parsley. Mix well and stir-fry for about five minutes.

Now add the lentils, 1 bay leaf, some salt and chili powder. Add about 4 cups of water and bring it to a boil. Reduce the heat, cover and cook until the lentils soften.

Sprinkle with some parsley before serving.

Nutrition information per serving: Kcal: 313, Protein: 36g, Carbs: 42g, Fats: 28g

19.   Breakfast Creamy Mozzarella Tricolore

Ingredients:

2 large tomatoes, sliced

3.5oz mozzarella, sliced

1 medium-sized avocado, halved and stone removed

3 tbsp of extra virgin olive oil

½ tsp of salt

1 tsp of apple cider vinegar

½ tsp of dried thyme, crushed

½ tsp of stevia

Preparation:

Wash and slice tomatoes. Place them on a serving platter.

Cut avocado in half and remove the stone. Slice thinly and make a layer over tomatoes. Top with mozzarella.

In a small bowl, whisk together olive oil, apple cider, thyme, salt, and stevia. Drizzle over tricolore and serve.

Nutrition information per serving: Kcal: 340 Protein: 16.5g, Carbs: 5.8g, Fats: 31g

20.   Warm Strawberry Coconut Flakes

Ingredients:

¼ cup of flaked coconut, lightly toasted

1 cup of almond milk (you can use coconut almond milk for some extra flavor)

1 tbsp of chia seeds

1 tbsp of almonds, minced

1 tbsp of coconut oil

1 tsp of strawberry extract, sugar-free

½ tsp of stevia

Preparation:

Preheat the oven to 350 degrees. Line some baking paper over a baking sheet and grease with melted coconut oil.

Pour the flakes onto the sheet and toast for 10-15 minutes. Remove from the oven and transfer to a bowl.

Add almond milk, minced almonds, chia seeds, strawberry extract, and stevia. Give it a good stir and serve warm.

Nutritional information per serving: Kcal: 175 , Protein: 3.1g, Carbs: 8.6g, Fats: 19g

21.   Baked Zucchini with Blue Cheese Drizzle

Ingredients:

1 medium-sized zucchini, sliced lengthwise

2 large eggs

¼ cup of almond milk

½ cup of almond flour

2 garlic cloves, crushed

1 tsp of dried oregano, crushed

½ cup of gorgonzola

1 tsp of salt

½ tsp of pepper

¼ cup of extra virgin olive oil

Preparation:

Preheat the oven to 350 degrees. Grease a quarter-sized sheet pan with some olive oil and set aside.

Combine the remaining oil with crushed garlic, oregano, and pepper. Set aside.

Slice the zucchini lengthwise and sprinkle with some salt. Set aside for 5-7 minutes. Rinse well and pat dry. Arrange a single layer in a baking dish. Using a kitchen brush, spread the olive oil mixture over each zucchini slice and bake for 20 minutes.

Meanwhile, whisk together eggs, almond milk, and almond flour. Beat well with an electric mixer on high until well incorporated. Spread this mixture over zucchini and continue to cook for five more minutes.

Place gorgonzola in a microwave for two minutes. Drizzle over zucchini and serve warm.

Nutritional information per serving: Kcal: 340, Protein: 19g, Carbs: 7.3g, Fats: 35g

22. Garlic Shiitake Casserole

Ingredients:

1lb shiitake mushrooms, whole

6 eggs

2 medium onions, peeled

3 garlic cloves, crushed

¼ cup of olive oil

½ tsp of sea salt

¼ tsp of freshly ground black pepper

Preparation:

Preheat the oven to 350 degrees. Spread 2 tbsp of olive oil over an eighth-sized baking sheet. Place the shiitake on a baking sheet. Bake for about 10-12 minutes. Remove from the oven and allow it to cool for a while. Lover the oven heat to 200 degrees.

Meanwhile, peel and finely chop the onions. Separate egg whites from yolks. Slice shiitake into ½ inch thick slices and place in a bowl. Add chopped onions, olive oil, egg whites, crushed garlic, salt and pepper. Mix well.

Spread this mixture over a baking sheet and bake for another 15-20 minutes.

Nutritional information per serving: Kcal: 319, Protein: 41g, Carbs: 14g, Fats: 34g

23.   Sweet Asparagus with Parmesan Cheese

Ingredients:

1lb fresh asparagus, woody ends trimmed

2 medium onions, peeled and finely chopped

2 small jalapeno peppers, sliced

1 cup of vegetable stock

¼ cup of fresh lime juice

1 tsp of pure orange extract, sugar-free

5 tbsp of extra virgin olive oil

1 tsp of dried rosemary, crushed

Preparation:

Heat up the olive oil in a large saucepan. Add chopped onions and stir-fry for 2-3 minutes, or until translucent.

Place jalapeno peppers, lime juice, orange extract, and rosemary in a food processor. Add about ½ cup of vegetable stock and pulse until smooth. Pour the mixture into a frying pan and reduce the heat to minimum. Simmer for ten minutes.

When most of the liquid has evaporated, add trimmed asparagus and the remaining vegetable stock. Bring it to a boil and simmer until asparagus are fork tender.

Serve warm.

Nutritional information per serving: Kcal: 180, Protein: 4.9g, Carbs: 7g, Fats: 41g

24.   Stripped Vegetables in Wok

Ingredients:

1 pound of button mushrooms, sliced

1 medium red bell pepper, cut into strips

1 medum green bell pepper, cut into strips

7-8 cauliflower florets

½ cup of parmesan cheese

7-8 brussel sprouts, halved

1 tbsp fresh tomato sauce, sugar-free

1 fire-roasted tomato, roughly chopped

1 tsp of salt

4 tbsp of extra virgin olive oil

Preparation:

Thoroughly wash and slice mushrooms lengthwise.

In a large wok pan, heat up the olive oil over a medium-high temperature. Add cauliflower florets and brussel sprouts and cook for ten minutes, stirring constantly. Now add stripped peppers, fire-roasted tomato, salt, tomato sauce, and parmesan cheese. Give it a good stir and cook for ten more minutes.

Now you can add mushrooms and continue to cook for 5-7 more minutes. Give it a final stir and serve warm.

Nutritional information per serving: Kcal: 313, Protein: 18.9g, Carbs: 14g, Fats: 32g

25.   Hot Chili Cauliflower Stew

Ingredients:

2 pounds of cauliflower florets

1 tbsp chili pepper, ground

1 tablespoon of vegetable oil

6 oz tomato paste, sugar-free

2 jalapeno peppers, cut into strips

1 large tomato, roughly chopped

1 large onion, peeled and finely chopped

1 cup of fresh button mushrooms, sliced

¼ tbsp of salt

1 bay leaf

2 ½ cups vegetable broth

1 tsp of dry thyme

3 garlic cloves, crushed

Preparation:

Take a frying pan and set it over high heat. Heat up the

vegetable oil and add the cauliflower florets to it. Cook, stirring constantly, until properly brown. Transfer to a deep pot. In the same pan, fry the onions, turning the heat to medium. Cook the onions for 5 minutes.

Now add jalapeno peppers, tomato paste, chili pepper, garlic and salt. Continue to cook for 3-4 minutes. Transfer to a pot.

Add the remaining ingredients and cover with a lid. Set the heat to minimum and cook for one hour.

Nutritional information per serving: Kcal: 180, Protein: 13g, Carbs: 25g, Fats: 8.9g

26.   Crustless Creamy Spinach Pie

Ingredients:

1 pack (9 ounces) of fresh spinach, chopped

4 whole eggs

½ cup of coconut milk

2 oz of crumbled Feta cheese

¼ cup grated Parmesan cheese

½ cup shredded Mozzarella cheese

3 tbsp of vegetable oil

1 tsp of salt

½ tsp of black pepper

Preparation:

Preheat the oven to 350°F. Lightly grease a baking dish with vegetable oil and set aside.

Whisk the eggs thoroughly in a mixing bowl. Gradually whisk in the milk and beat well on high. Add parmesan and continue to beat until well combined. Set aside.

Place the chopped spinach in the greased baking dish and add crumbled Feta cheese. Pour in the egg mixture and cover the other ingredients completely.

Bake for about 40 to 45 minutes or until the cheese has melted and lightly browned.

Remove from the oven and chill for 10-15 minutes before serving.

Nutritional information per serving: Kcal: 190, Protein: 15g, Carbs: 8g, Fats: 20g

27. Lamb's Lettuce with Fresh Goat's Cheese and Tomatoes

Ingredients:

5 cherry tomatoes, whole

A handful of black olives

1 medium-sized onion, peeled and sliced

3.5 oz fresh goat's cheese

2 radishes, sliced

3.5 oz of lamb's lettuce

2 tbsp of freshly squeezed lime juice

3 tbsp of extra virgin olive oil

Salt to taste

Preparation:

Place the vegetables in a large bowl. Add olive oil, goat's cheese, fresh lime juice and some salt to taste. Toss to combine.

Nutritional information per serving: Kcal: 225, Protein: 18.5g, Carbs: 10g, Fats: 35g

28.   Cheesy Button Mushrooms

Ingredients:

2 small zucchinis, sliced lengthwise

½ cup of cottage cheese

1 cup of lamb's lettuce

1 cup of cherry tomatoes

½ cup of button mushrooms, sliced

1 tsp of salt

½ tsp of freshly ground black pepper

2 tbsp of olive oil

Preparation:

Wash and pat dry the zucchini with some kitchen paper. Slice lengthwise.

Use a large grill pan and grease it with some olive oil. Heat up over medium-high heat and sliced zucchinis. Grill for 3-4 minutes on each side, remove from the heat and chill for a while.

Meanwhile add mushrooms into the grill pan and grill until the liquid evaporates. Remove from the heat and chill for a while.

Place lamb's lettuce, cottage cheese, and cherry tomatoes in a large bowl. Add grilled zucchini, mushrooms, and season with salt and pepper. Toss to combine and serve.

Nutritional information per serving: Kcal: 220, Protein: 27g, Carbs: 14g, Fats: 24g

29.   Vegge Cabbage Rolls

Ingredients:

1 pound of fresh cabbage leaves

3 large eggs

½ cup of cauliflower, pre-cooked and finely chopped

1 medium-sized tomato

1 tbsp of fresh parsley, chopped

¼ tsp of sea salt

¼ tsp of black pepper, ground

5 tbsp of olive oil

Preparation:

Gently place the eggs in a deep pot. Add enough water to cover and bring it to a boil. Cook for 10 minutes. Remove from the heat, cool for a while and peel. Place in a medium-sized bowl and mash with a fork. Set aside.

Wash, peel and finely chop the tomato. Place it in a large bowl. Combine the eggs, chopped cauliflower, parsley, salt, and pepper. Add about two tablespoons of olive oil to this mixture. Place about two tablespoons of this mixture in the center of each cabbage leaf. Roll up nicely tuck in the ends.

Now add the remaining oil in a deep pot. Carefully place the rolls in a pot and add about 1 cup of water. Cover and cook over a medium-high heat for about 20 minutes.

Nutritional information per serving: Kcal: 240, Protein: 29g, Carbs: 27g, Fats: 42g

30.   Warm Broccoli Slaw

Ingredients:

12 oz bag broccoli slaw

½ cup of brussel sprouts, halved

½ cup of cauliflower, chopped

A hanful of finely chopped kale

3 tbsp of sesame oil

1 tsp of ginger, grated

½ tsp of salt

¼ cup of goat milk yogurt

Preparation:

Heat up the oil in a large skillet. Add brussel sprouts and chopped cauliflower. Cook for 10-15 minutes, stirring constantly.

Stir in brocoli slaw, grated ginger, salt, and kale. Add about ¼ cup of water and continue to cook for another 10 minutes. When the water has evaporated, stir in yogurt and remove from the heat.

Serve warm.

Nutritional information per serving: Kcal: 214, Protein: 9g, Carbs: 13g, Fats: 15g

31.   Vegetarian Kebab

Ingredients:

1 lb rib cauliflower florets, halved

2 large onions, grated

5 tbsp of extra virgin olive oil

½ tsp of red pepper, crushed

½ tsp of dried oregano

¼ tsp of salt

¼ tsp of ground black pepper

1 tbsp of tomato sauce

2 cups of lukewarm water

1 large tomato, sliced into wedges

½ green pepper, chopped

1 cup of plain yogurt, or sour cream

Preparation:

First, put the onions into a blender and blend until smooth. Transfer the liquid from the blender into a large bowl, and remove the remaining pulp.

Cut the cauliflower florets and slice it into bite-sized pieces.

Combine the spices with two tablespoons of olive oil and onions. Stir well. Now add the cauliflower and stir all together. Cover the lid and set aside.

Now, preheat the remaining olive oil over a medium temperature. Add the tomato sauce and stir well. If you're a fan of spicy food, you can add a pinch of crushed chili pepper. This, however, is optional. Now add the water, a pinch of salt, and gently simmer for a couple of minutes. Remove from the heat and set aside.

Meanwhile, heat up 2 tablespoons of vegetable oil and add the cauliflower. Stir-fry for about ten minutes. Now add the tomato sauce and onions. Stir well and cook for another five minutes. Set aside.

Place the cauliflower pieces onto a serving platter, top with tomato and pepper, and serve with some yogurt or sour cream.

Enjoy!

Nutritional information per serving: Kcal: 190, Protein: 12g, Carbs: 21g, Fats: 22g

32. Cold Gazpacho

Ingredients:

1 pound of fresh tomatoes, peeled and finely chopped

3 large cucumbers, finely chopped

3 spring onions, finely chopped

1 medium-sized red onion, finely chopped

1 tbsp of tomato paste, sugar-free

½ tsp of salt

1 tbsp of ground cumin

¼ tsp of pepper

Fresh parsley, for serving

Preparation:

Preheat the non-stick frying pan over a medium-high temperature. Add the onions and stir-fry for 3-4 minutes. Now add the tomatoes, tomato paste, cucumber, cumin, salt, and pepper. Cook for another five minutes, or until caramelized.

Add three cups of lukewarm water, reduce the heat to minimum and cook for about 15 minutes. Now add about

1 cup of water and bring it to a boil. Remove from the heat and serve with fresh parsley.

Serve cold.

Nutritional information per serving: Kcal: 320, Protein: 12.5g, Carbs: 70g, Fats: 13g

33.   Sweet Almond Patties

Ingredients:

1lb cauliflower florets, sliced

7oz almonds, toasted

1 cup of almond milk

1 egg

1 tsp of sea salt

1 tbsp of almond butter

1 cup of almond flour

½ cup of parsley, finely chopped

½ cup of plain yougurt

Vegetable oil

Preparation:

Place cauliflower florets in a deep pot. Add enough water to cover and bring it to a boil. Cook until fork tender. Remove from the heat and transfer to a bowl. Add one teaspoon of salt, almond milk, and almond butter. Mash until a smooth puree. Set aside.

Finely chop the almonds and combine with cauliflower puree. Add almond flour, eggs, and parsley. Mix until well combined. Using your hands, shape 1-inch thick patties.

Preheat some oil over a medium-high heat. Fry each patty for about 2-3 minutes on each side.

Nutritional information per serving: Kcal: 322, Protein: 17g, Carbs: 18g, Fats: 28g

34.   Creamy Cheese Lettuce Wraps

Ingredients:

3 large iceberg lettuce leaves

1 medium-sized tomato

½ red bell pepper, finely chopped

1 garlic clove, crushed

1 tsp of dry oregano

2 tbsp of grated goat's cheese (can be replaced with some other cheese)

1 tsp of extra virgin olive oil

½ tsp of salt

2 tbsp of finely chopped parsley

Preparation:

Combine together tomato, chopped pepper, crushed garlic clove, oregano, olive oil, salt, and parsley in a large bowl. Spread some of the mixture over each lettuce leaf and wrap. Secure with a toothpick and serve.

Enjoy!

Nutritional information per serving: Kcal: 133, Protein: 7g, Carbs: 11g, Fats: 21g

35. Braised Greens with Fresh Mint

Ingredients:

3.5oz fresh chicory, torn

3.5oz wild asparagus, finely chopped

3.5oz Swiss chard, torn

A handful of fresh mint, chopped

A handful of rocket salad, torn

3 garlic cloves, crushed

¼ tsp of freshly ground black pepper

1 tsp of salt

¼ cup of fresh lemon juice

Olive oil

Preparation:

Fill a large pot with salted water and add greens. Bring it to a boil and cook for 2-3 minutes. Remove from the heat and drain.

In a medium-sized skillet, heat up 3 tablespoons of olive oil. Add crushed garlic and stir-fry for about 2-3 minutes. Now add the greens, salt, pepper, and about half of the lemon juice. Stir-fry the greens for five more minutes.

Remove from the heat. Season with more lemon juice and serve.

Nutritional information per serving: Kcal: 55, Protein: 4g, Carbs: 7g, Fats: 8g

36.   Warm Caponata

Ingredients:

7oz brussel sprouts, chopped into bite sized pieces

1 zucchini, sliced

1 medium-sized onion, peeled and chopped

2 large, fresh tomatoes, roughly chopped

3.5 oz cabbage, shredded

1 medium-sized chili pepper

2 stalks of celery

3 tbsp of olive oil

1 tbsp of red wine vinegar

Salt to taste

1 tsp of stevia

½ tbsp of basil, dry

Preparation:

Chop zucchini into bite-sized pieces and season with some salt. Allow it to stand for about 5 minutes and rinse well.

Meanwhile, heat up the olive oil over a medium heat. Add the onions and stir-fry for 2-3 minutes. Now add celery, basil, stevia, salt, vinegar, and tomatoes. Continue to cook for 2 more minutes.

Transfer to a deep pot and add other ingredients. Add about one cup of water and cook for about 20 minutes over high temperature.

Nutritional information per serving: Kcal: 160, Protein: 11g, Carbs: 28g, Fats: 9g

37.   Creamy Manicotti

Ingredients:

5 crepes

¼ cup of coconut oil

3oz coconut flour

2pts coconut milk

8.8oz ricotta cheese

3oz grated Parmesan cheese

5oz fresh spinach, torn

Seasoning to taste

Preparation:

Preheat the oven to 350 degrees.

Bring the coconut oil, flour and milk slowly to a boil, whisking constantly until thickened. Put half of the sauce into a bowl and mix with ricotta, parmesan, spinach, and seasoning to taste.

Lay a crepe on the work surface. Spoon out about 1/5 of the mixture and place it on crepe. Roll up the crepe and place it on a baking sheet. Repeat the process until you have used all the ingredients.

Bake for 10 minutes, remove from the oven and serve.

Nutritional information per serving: Kcal: 500, Protein: 31g, Carbs: 11.5g, Fats: 50g

38.   Sweet tomato soup

Ingredients:

2oz tomato, peeled and roughly chopped

Ground black pepper to taste

1 tbsp of celery, finely chopped

1 onion, diced

1 tbsp of fresh basil, finely chopped

Fresh water

Preparation:

Preheat the non-stick frying pan over a medium-high temperature. Add the onions, celery, and fresh basil. Sprinkle some pepper and stir-fry for about 10 minutes, until caramelized.

Add the tomato and about ¼ cup of water. Reduce the heat to minimum and cook for about 15 minutes, until softened. Now add about 1 cup of water and bring it to a boil. Remove from the heat and serve with fresh parsley.

Nutrition information per serving: Kcal: 25 Protein: 0.7g, Carbs: 4.9g, Fats: 0.9g

39. Chocolate Protein Bars

Ingredients:

1 cup of toasted almonds, finely chopped

½ cup of cocoa butter

½ cup of sweetener, powdered

2 tablespoons of chia seeds

¼ cup of raw cocoa powder

3 egg whites

¼ cup of coconut milk

Preparation:

Combine the ingredients in a bowl and mix well to combine. Shape the balls using your hands and refrigerate for about 30 minutes.

Nutritional information per serving: Kcal: 260, Protein: 11g, Carbs: 9g, Fats: 28g

40.   Chef salad to go

Ingredients:

3 large eggs

½ cucumber, sliced

1 small tomato, roughly chopped

1 cup of fresh lettuce, torn

1 small green pepper, sliced

½ tsp salt

1 tbsp of lime juice

3 tbsp of olive oil

Preparation:

Hard boil the eggs for 10 minutes. Remove from the heat, rinse and chill for a while. Gently peel and slice each egg. Transfer to a large jar.

Now, combine the vegetables in a glass jar. Add the meat and mix well. Season with salt and some lime juice. Seal the lid and you're ready to go.

Nutritional information per serving: Kcal: 55, Protein: 7g, Carbs: 2.8g, Fats: 11.3g

41.　Super Healthy Beet Greens Salad

Ingredients:

8 oz leek, chopped into bite-size pieces

Handful of beet greens

1 large tomato, chopped

2 garlic cloves, finely chopped

3 tbsp of vegetable oil

A few mint leaves

½ tsp of salt

½ tsp of red pepper

½ tsp of Cayenne pepper

Preparation:

Heat up some vegetable oil in a large skillet. Stir-fry the garlic for 2-3 minutes, or until lightly charred. Now add leek, salt, pepper, and cayenne pepper. Cook for ten minutes, over medium heat, stirring constantly. Remove from the heat and transfer to a bowl.

Add a handful of beet greens, chopped tomato, and fresh mint. Toss well to combine and serve.

Nutritional information per serving: Kcal: 133, Protein: 2.1g, Carbs: 15g, Fats: 15.5g

42.   Ginger Peach Smoothie

Ingredients:

1 cup of coconut milk

1 tbsp of coconut oil

1 tbsp of chia seeds

1 tsp of ginger, ground

2 tsp of sweetener, powdered

1 tsp of pure peach extract, sugar-free

Preparation:

Combine the ingredients in a blender and pulse to combine. You can add some ice cubes, but this is optional. Serve cold.

Nutritional information per serving: Kcal: 417, Protein: 6g, Carbs: 10g, Fats: 41g

43.   Cherry Avocado Smoothie

Ingredients:

½ ripe avocado, chopped

1 cup of coconut water, sugar-free

1 tbsp of fresh lime juice

1 tsp of sweetener, powdered

1 tsp of pure cherry extract, sugar-free

Preparation:

Place the ingredients in a food processor and pulse to combine. Serve cold.

Nutritional information per serving: Kcal: 210, Protein: 4.5g, Carbs: 18g, Fats: 16g

44.   Fresh Avocado Smoothie

Ingredients:

½ avocado, roughly chopped

1 cup of coconut milk

1 tbsp of walnuts, chopped

1 tsp of vanilla extract, sugar-free

1 tsp sweetener, powdered

A handful of ice cubes

Preparation:

Place the ingredients in a blender and pulse to combine. Serve cold.

Nutritional information per serving: Kcal: 212, Protein: 8g, Carbs: 12g, Fats: 36g

45. Coconut Yogurt with Chia Seeds and Almonds

Ingredients:

1 cup of coconut yogurt

3 tbsp of chia seeds

1 tsp of toasted almonds, finely chopped

2 tsp of sweetener, powdered

Preparation:

For this easy recipe, combine 3 tbsp of chia seeds with 1 cup of coconut yogurt, 1 tsp of ground almonds and 1 tbsp of honey. Use a fork or an electric mixer to get a smooth mixture. Allow it to cool in the refrigerator.

You can combine ¾ cup of coconut yogurt with ¼ cup of rice yogurt for extra flavor.

Nutritional information per serving: Kcal: 312, Protein: 14g, Carbs: 44g, Fats: 41g

46.   Coco Pudding

Ingredients:

2 cups of unsweetened coconut milk (you can use almond milk for extra flavor)

¼ cup of toasted coconut flakes

1 tbsp walnuts, finely chopped

1 tbps of hazelnuts, finely chopped

1 tsp of stevia, powdered

1 tsp of cinnamon, ground

½ tbsp of sugar-free vanilla extract

Preparation:

In a medium sized saucepan bring 2 cups of coconut milk to boil. Gently stir in the coconut flakes and reduce the heat to minimum. Cook until they double in size and then add walnuts, hazelnuts, stevia, cinnamon, and vanilla extract.

Give it a good stir and cook for five more minutes.

Remove from the heat and chill for a while. Transfer to serving bowls and cool in the refrigerator for about 30 minutes before serving.

Nutritional information per serving: Kcal: 193, Protein: 3.8g, Carbs: 6g, Fats: 12g

Juices

1.   Apple Beet Juice

Ingredients:

1 small apple, cored

1 cup of beets, sliced

1 whole kiwi, sliced

¼ tsp of ceylon cinnamon, ground

Preparation:

Wash the apple and remove the core and cut into bite-sized pieces.

Wash the beets and trim off the green ends. Peel and cut into thin slices. Fill the measuring cup.

Peel the kiwi and cut lengthwise in half. Set aside.

Now process apple, beets and kiwi in a juicer until well juiced or shake.

Transfer to a serving glass and stir in the ceylon cinnamon.

Refrigerate for 15 minutes before serving.

Enjoy!

Nutritional information per serving: Kcal: 139, Protein: 3.3g, Carbs: 40.6g, Fats: 0.7g

2.   Peach Plum Juice

Ingredients:

2 medium-sized peaches, pitted

2 whole plums, pitted

1 whole lemon, peeled

¼ tsp of ginger, ground

Preparation:

Wash the peaches and cut in half. Remove the pits and cut into bite-sized pieces. Set aside.

Wash the plums and cut lengthwise in half. Remove the pits and set aside.

Peel the lemons and cut lengthwise in half. Set aside.

Add ingredients into a juicer and stir thoroughly.

Transfer to a serving glass and stir in the ginger.

Nutritional information per serving: Kcal: 161, Protein: 4.2g, Carbs: 49.1g, Fats: 1.2g

3.   Peach Carrots Juice

Ingredients:

2 large peaches

10 medium sized carrots

2 large sized apples

1 large sized orange, peeled

½ of a lemon, skin peeled away

Preparation:

Wash the peaches and cut in half. Remove the pits and cut into bite-sized pieces. Set aside.

Wash the carrots and peel them. Cut into small chunks and set aside.

Wash the apple and remove the core and cut into bite-sized pieces.

Peel the orange and divide into wedges. Set aside.

Peel the lemon and cut lengthwise in half. Set aside.

Add ingredients into a juicer and stir thoroughly.

Transfer to a serving glass .

Refrigerate for 15 minutes before serving.

Enjoy!

Nutritional information per serving: Kcal: 139, Protein: 3.3g, Carbs: 40.6g, Fats: 0.7g

4.   Spinach Apple Green Juice

Ingredients:

1 cup of fresh spinach, chopped

1 medium-sized Granny Smith's apple, cored

1 cup of cucumber, sliced

1 small ginger knob, peeled

Preparation:

Wash the spinach thoroughly under cold running water. Slightly drain and chop into small pieces. Set aside.

Wash the apple and cut in half. Remove the core and cut into small chunks. Set aside.

Wash the cucumber and cut into thin slices. Fill the measuring cup and reserve the rest for later.

Peel the ginger and set aside.

Combine all ingredients within a juicer and enjoy this super tasty and health boosting green juice drink

Transfer to a serving glass and stir in the salt.

Serve immediately.

Nutritional information per serving: Kcal: 126, Protein: 3.6g, Carbs: 35.8g, Fats: 0.8g

5.   Kiwi Mango Juice

Ingredients:

1 whole kiwi, peeled

1 cup of mango, chunked

1 cup of fresh spinach, chopped

1 small ginger knob, peeled

Preparation:

Peel the kiwi and cut lengthwise in half. Set aside.

Peel the mango and cut into small chunks. Fill the measuring cup and reserve the rest in the refrigerator.

Wash the spinach thoroughly under cold running water. Slightly drain and chop it into small pieces. Set aside.

Peel the ginger knob and set aside.

Now, combine mango, kiwi, spinach, and ginger in a juicer and process until juiced.

Transfer to a serving glass.

Refrigerate for 10 minutes before serving.

Enjoy!

Nutritional information per serving: Kcal: 190, Protein: 9.1g, Carbs: 53.6g, Fats: 2.2g

6.   Apple Avocado Asparagus Juice

Ingredients:

1 small Golden Delicious apple, cored

1 cup of avocado, cubed

1 cup of fresh asparagus, trimmed

1 whole lime, peeled

1 small ginger knob, peeled

Preparation:

Wash the apple and cut in half. Remove the core and cut into small chunks. Set aside.

Peel the avocado and cut lengthwise in half. Remove the pit and cut into small chunks. Set aside.

Wash the asparagus and trim off the woody ends. Cut into bite-sized pieces and set aside.

Peel the lime and cut lengthwise in half. Set aside.

Peel the ginger knob and cut into small pieces. Set aside.

Now, process apple, avocado, asparagus, lime and ginger in a juicer.

Transfer to a serving glass.

Refrigerate for 15 minutes before serving.

Enjoy!

Nutritional information per serving: Kcal: 298, Protein: 7.3g, Carbs: 41.6g, Fats: 22.5g

7.   Mango Cantaloupe Juice

Ingredients:

1 cup of mango, chunked

1 cup of cantaloupe, diced

1 medium-sized peach, pitted

1 whole lime, peeled

¼ tsp of ceylon cinnamon, ground

Preparation:

Wash and peel the mango. Cut into small chunks and set aside.

Cut the cantaloupe in half. Scoop out the seeds and cut two wedges and peel them. Chop into chunks and set aside. Reserve the rest of the cantaloupe in a refrigerator.

Wash the peach and cut lengthwise in half. Remove the pit and cut into bite-sized pieces. Set aside.

Peel the lime and cut lengthwise in half. Set aside.

Now, combine mango, cantaloupe, peach and lime in a juicer. Process until well juiced.

Transfer to a serving glass and stir in the ceylon cinnamon.

Serve immediately.

Enjoy!

Nutritional information per serving: Kcal: 205, Protein: 5.2g, Carbs: 59.2g, Fats: 1.6g

8.   Avocado Strawberry Juice

Ingredients:

1 cup of avocado, cubed

1 cup of strawberries, chopped

1 cup of cucumber, sliced

1 medium-sized orange, wedged

1 cup of Swiss chard

Preparation:

Peel the avocado and cut in half. Remove the pit and cut into cubes. Fill the measuring cup and reserve the rest for later

Wash the strawberries and cut into small pieces. Set aside.

Wash the cucumber and cut into thin slices. Fill the measuring cup and reserve the rest for later.

Peel the orange and divide into wedges. Chop each wedge in half and set aside.

Wash the Swiss chard under cold running water. Slightly drain and roughly chop it. Set aside.

Now, combine avocado, strawberries, cucumber, orange,

and Swiss chard in a juicer. Process until well juiced.

Transfer to a serving glass and add some crushed ice before serving.

Enjoy!

Nutritional information per serving: Kcal: 241, Protein: 4.24g, Carbs: 26.54g, Fats: 21.62g

9. Avocado Fennel Juice

Ingredients:

1 cup of avocado, chunked

1 cup of fennel, chopped

1 small Granny Smith's apple, chopped

1 cup of cucumber, sliced

¼ tsp of ginger, ground

Preparation:

Peel the avocado and cut in half. Remove the pit and cut into small chunks. Fill the measuring cup and reserve the rest for later.

Wash the fennel bulb and trim off the wilted outer layers. Cut into small chunks and fill the measuring cup. Reserve the rest in the refrigerator.

Wash the apple and remove the core. Cut into bite-sized pieces and set aside.

Wash the cucumber and cut into thin slices. Fill the measuring cup and reserve the rest in the refrigerator. Set aside.

Now, combine avocado, fennel, apple, and cucumber in a juicer and process until juiced.

Transfer to a serving glass and stir in the ginger.

Add some ice before serving.

Enjoy!

Nutritional information per serving: Kcal: 286, Protein: 5g, Carbs: 40.3g, Fats: 21.9g

10.   Blueberry Watermelon Juice

Ingredients:

2 cups of blueberries

1 cup of watermelon, cubed

1 cup of fresh basil, torn

1 oz of water

Preparation:

Place the blueberries in a large colander. Rinse well under cold running water and set aside.

Cut one large watermelon wedge. Using a sharp paring knife, peel and cut into small cubes. Remove the seeds and set aside.

Wash the basil and roughly torn it with hands. Set aside.

Now, combine blueberries, watermelon, and basil in a juicer. Process until juiced.

Transfer to a serving glass and stir in the water.

Refrigerate for 10 minutes before serving.

Nutritional information per serving: Kcal: 188, Protein: 3.8g, Carbs: 55g, Fats: 1.3g

11.   Blueberry Spinach Juice

Ingredients:

2 cups of fresh spinach, chopped

1 cup of cucumber, sliced

1 Apple, cored

1 Big Handful Blueberries

2 Carrots

¼ tsp of ginger, ground

Preparation:

Wash the spinach thoroughly under cold running water. Slightly drain and chop into small pieces. Set aside.

Wash the cucumber and cut into thin slices. Fill the measuring cup and reserve the rest for later.

Wash the apple and remove the core and cut into bite-sized pieces.

Place the blueberries in a large colander. Rinse well under cold running water and set aside.

Wash and peel the carrots. Cut into thin slices and fill the measuring cup. Reserve the rest in the refrigerator.

Now, combine spinach, cucumber, apple, blueberries and carrots in a juicer. Process until juiced.

Transfer to a serving glass and stir in the ginger.

Serve immediately.

Enjoy!

Nutritional information per serving: Kcal: 203, Protein: 4.8g, Carbs: 60.5g, Fats: 1.3g

12.   Beet Orange Juice

Ingredients:

1 whole beet, sliced

1 medium-sized orange, peeled

1 cup of cucumber, sliced

1 tbsp of liquid honey

Preparation:

Wash the beet and trim off the green parts. Cut into thin slices and set aside.

Peel the orange and divide into wedges. Cut each wedge in half and set aside.

Wash the cucumber and cut into thin slices. Fill the measuring cup and reserve the rest in the refrigerator.

Now, combine beet, orange and cucumber in a juicer and process until juiced. Transfer to a serving glass and stir in the honey.

Serve immediately.

Enjoy!

Nutritional information per serving: Kcal: 83, Protein: 2.8g, Carbs: 25.1g, Fats: 0.3g

13.   Green Juice

Ingredients:

4 cups of fresh spinach,chopped

4 medium green Granny Smith's apples, cored

¼ cup of fresh mint leaves,torn

3 large kale leaves,torn

3 large stalks of celery, chopped

1 ½ cup of fresh basil,torn

Preparation:

Wash the spinach thoroughly under cold running water. Chop into small pieces and fill the measuring cup. Reserve the rest for later.

Wash the apple and cut lengthwise in half. Remove the core and cut into bite-sized pieces. Set aside.

Combine kale and mint in a large colander. Wash thoroughly under cold running water. Slightly drain and torn with hands. Set aside.

Wash the celery stalk and cut into small pieces. Set aside.

Wash the basil and roughly torn it with hands. Set aside.

Place all ingredients through a juicer and blend together.Process until juiced.

Refrigerate for 10 minutes before serving.

Enjoy!

Nutritional information per serving: Kcal: 425, Protein: 17.2g, Carbs: 122.2g Fats: 4.1g

14.   Carrot Plum Juice

Ingredients:

4 whole plum, chopped

1 cup of carrots, sliced

1 cup of Romaine lettuce, shredded

1 cup of mustard greens, torn

1 oz of water

Preparation:

Wash the plums and cut each in half. Remove the pits and set aside.

Wash and peel the carrots. Cut into thin slices and fill the measuring cup. Reserve the rest in the refrigerator.

Combine lettuce and mustard greens in a large colander. Rinse well under cold running water. Shred the lettuce torn the mustard greens using hands. Set aside.

Now, combine carrots, plums, lettuce, and mustard greens in a juicer and process until juiced. Transfer to a serving glass and stir in the water.

Serve cold.

Nutritional information per serving: Kcal: 128, Protein: 4.8g, Carbs: 39.1g, Fats: 1.3g

15.   Avocado Raspberry Juice

Ingredients:

1 cup of avocado, chunked

1 cup of raspberries

1 small peach, pitted

3 whole apricots, chopped

¼ tsp of ceylon cinnamon, ground

Preparation:

Peel the avocado and cut lengthwise in half. Cut into thin slices and reserve the rest in the refrigerator. Set aside.

Wash the raspberries using a colander. Slightly drain and fill the measuring cup. Reserve the rest in the refrigerator or freezer for later.

Wash the peach and cut in half. Remove the pit and cut into bite-sized pieces. Set aside.

Wash the apricots and cut in half. Remove the pits and cut in quarters. Set aside.

Now, combine avocado, raspberries, peach, and apricots in a juicer and process until juiced.

Transfer to a serving glass and stir in the ceylon cinnamon.

Refrigerate for 15 minutes before serving.

Enjoy!

Nutritional information per serving: Kcal: 206, Protein: 5.5g, Carbs: 63.5g, Fats: 2.1g

16. Celery Kale Juice

Ingredients:

2 medium-sized celery stalk, chopped

1 cup of fresh kale, chopped

1 small apple, cored

1 cup of Romaine lettuce, shredded

1 ½ cup of fresh basil,torn

Preparation:

Wash the celery stalks and cut into bite-sized pieces. Set aside

Wash the kale thoroughly under cold running water. Slightly drain and chop it into small pieces. Set aside.

Wash the apple and cut in half. Remove the core and cut into small pieces. Set aside.

Wash the lettuce leaves and shred it. Fill the measuring cup and reserve the rest for later.

Wash the basil and roughly torn it with hands. Set aside.

Now, combine kale, celery, apple, lettuce and basil in a juicer and process until juiced.

Transfer to a serving glass and add some ice before serving.

Enjoy!

Nutritional information per serving: Kcal: 103, Protein: 4.6g, Carbs: 29.4g, Fats: 1.2g

17.   Spinach Cauliflower Juice

Ingredients:

2 cup of fresh spinach, torn

5 cauliflower flowerets, chopped

2 cup of black grapes

1 oz of water

¼ tsp of ginger, ground

Preparation:

Wash the spinach thoroughly under running water. Torn with hands and set aside.

Wash the cauliflower flowerets and chop into small pieces. Fill the measuring cup and reserve the rest for later.

Wash the grapes and fill the measuring cup. Reserve the rest for later.

Now, combine cauliflower, spinach and grapes in a juicer and process until juiced.

Transfer to a serving glass and stir in the water and ginger.

Add some ice and serve immediately.

Enjoy!

Nutritional information per serving: Kcal: 136, Protein: 4.1g, Carbs: 36.9g, Fats: 1g

18.   Grape Blueberry Juice

Ingredients:

1 cup of black grapes

1 cup of blueberries

1 small Golden Delicious apple, cored

¼ tsp of cinnamon, ground

Preparation:

Wash the grapes and fill the measuring cup. Reserve the rest for later.

Wash the blueberries using a colander. Slightly drain and set aside.

Wash the apple and cut in half. Remove the core and cut into bite-sized pieces. Set aside.

Now, combine grapes, blueberries and apple in a juicer and process until juiced.

Transfer to a serving glass and stir in the cinnamon.

Add some ice before serving.

Enjoy!

Nutritional information per serving: Kcal: 191, Protein: 2.1g, Carbs: 54.7g, Fats: 1g

19.   Blueberry Grapes Juice

Ingredients:

2 cups of blueberries

1 cup of black grapes

1 medium-sized blood orange, peeled

1 small ginger knob, peeled and chopped

Preparation:

Place the blueberries in a colander. Wash thoroughly under cold running water and drain. Fill the measuring cups and reserve the rest in the freezer.

Wash the grapes and fill the measuring cup. Set aside.

Peel the orange and divide into wedges. Cut each wedge in half and set aside.

Peel the ginger and cut into small pieces. Set aside.

Now, combine blueberries, grapes, orange and ginger in a juicer and process until juiced.

Transfer to a serving glass and add few ice cubes before serving.

Enjoy!

Nutritional information per serving: Kcal: 254, Protein: 4.1g, Carbs: 75.2g, Fats: 1.5g

20.   Kiwi Broccoli Juice

Ingredients:

1 whole kiwi, sliced

1 cup of broccoli, chopped

1 medium-sized Granny Smith's apple, cored

1 medium-sized celery stalk, cut into bite-sized pieces

1 cup of fresh spinach, chopped

1 small ginger knob, peeled and chopped

Preparation:

Peel the kiwi and cut lengthwise in half. Set aside.

Wash the broccoli and chop into small pieces. Set aside.

Wash the apple and cut in half. Remove the core and cut into small chunks. Set aside.

Wash the celery and cut into bite-sized pieces. Set aside.

Wash the spinach thoroughly under cold running water. Chop into small pieces and fill the measuring cup. Reserve the rest for later.

Peel the ginger knob and chop it into small pieces. Set

aside.

Now, combine kiwi, broccoli, apple, celery, spinach and ginger in a juicer and process until well juiced.

Transfer to serving glass and add some ice before serving.

Enjoy!

Nutritional information per serving: Kcal: 146, Protein: 1.2g, Carbs: 42.2g, Fats: 1.2g

21.   Artichoke Spinach Juice

Ingredients:

1 medium-sized artichoke, chopped

1 cup of fresh spinach, chopped

2 cup of black grapes

1 Big Handful Blueberries

1 small ginger knob, peeled and sliced

Preparation:

Trim off the outer leaves of the artichoke using a sharp paring knife. Wash it and cut into bite-sized pieces. Set aside.

Using a colander, rinse the spinach thoroughly under cold running water. Chop into small pieces and set aside.

Wash the grapes and fill the measuring cup. Reserve the rest for later.

Place the blueberries in a large colander. Rinse well under cold running water and set aside.

Peel the ginger knob and chop it into small pieces. Set aside.

Now, combine artichoke, spinach, black grapes, blueberries and ginger in a juicer and process until juiced.

Transfer to a serving glass and refrigerate for 10 minutes before serving.

Enjoy!

Nutritional information per serving: Kcal: 229, Protein: 7.4g, Carbs: 68.6g, Fats: 1.4g

22.   Cabbage Avocado Juice

Ingredients:

1 cup of avocado, sliced

1 cup of purple cabbage, chopped

1 whole leek, chopped

1 medium-sized pear, chopped

½ lime, peeled

Preparation:

Peel the avocado and cut lengthwise in half. Cut into thin slices and reserve the rest in the refrigerator. Set aside.

Wash the cabbage thoroughly and chop into small pieces. Set aside.

Wash the leek and cut into bite-sized pieces. Set aside.

Wash the pear and remove the core. Cut into bite-sized pieces and set aside.

Peel the lime and cut lengthwise in half. Set aside.

Now, combine avocado, cabbage, leek, pear and lime in a juicer and process until juiced.

Transfer to a serving glass and refrigerate for 15 minutes before serving.

Enjoy!

Nutritional information per serving: Kcal: 352, Protein: 6.35g, Carbs: 62.41g, Fats: 22.09g

23. Red Juice

Ingredients:

2 leaves of purple cabbage, chopped

2 medium-sized Red Delicious apple, cored

3 medium-sized carrot, sliced

1 cup of strawberries, sliced

¼ beet, sliced

Preparation:

Wash the cabbage thoroughly and chop into small pieces. Set aside.

Wash the apple and cut in half. Remove the core and cut into small chunks. Set aside.

Wash and peel carrots. Cut into thin slices and set aside.

Wash the strawberries and remove the stems. Cut into small pieces and fill the measuring cup. Set aside.

Wash the beets and trim off the green parts. Cut into bite-sized pieces and set aside.

Now, combine cabbage, apple, carrot, strawberries and beet in a juicer and process until juiced.

Transfer to a serving glass and refrigerate for 10 minutes before serving.

Enjoy!

Nutritional information per serving: Kcal: 302, Protein: 5.2g, Carbs: 88.6g, Fats: 1.4g

24.   Cauliflower Beet greens Juice

Ingredients:

1 cup of cauliflower, chopped

1 cup of beet greens, torn

1 cup of fresh basil, torn

1 medium-sized red apple, cored

1 large lemon, peeled

1 cup of broccoli, chopped

Preparation:

Trim off the outer leaves of a cauliflower. Wash it and fill and cut into small pieces. Fill the measuring cup and reserve the rest in the refrigerator.

Combine beet greens and basil in a large colander. Rinse under cold running water and drain. Torn with hands and set aside.

Wash the apple and cut lengthwise in half. Remove the core and cut into bite-sized pieces. Set aside.

Peel the lemon and cut lengthwise in half. Set aside.

Wash the broccoli and chop into small pieces. Set aside.

Now, combine cauliflower, beet greens, basil, apple, lemon and broccoli, in a juicer. Process until well juiced and transfer to a serving glass.

Add few ice cubes and serve immediately.

Enjoy!

Nutritional information per serving: Kcal: 137, Protein: 7.3g, Carbs: 42.1g, Fats: 1.3g

25. Beet Orange Juice

Ingredients:

2 large beets, trimmed and chopped

1 large orange, wedged

1 cup of broccoli, chopped

1 large cucumber, sliced

Preparation:

Wash the beets and trim off the green parts. Cut into bite-sized pieces and set aside.

Peel the orange and divide into wedges. Set aside.

Wash the broccoli and cut into bite-sized pieces. Fill the measuring cup and reserve the rest for later.

Wash the cucumber and cut into thin slices. Set aside.

Now, combine beets, orange, broccoli, and cucumber in a juicer and process until juiced.

Garnish with some fresh mint, if you like.

Transfer to a serving glass and add some ice before serving.

Enjoy!

Nutritional information per serving: Kcal: 123, Protein: 7.8g, Carbs: 38.1g, Fats: 1.1g

26.   Cauliflower Kale Juice

Ingredients:

1 cup of cauliflower, chopped

1 cup of fresh kale, torn

1 cup of broccoli, chopped

1 small green apple, cored

¼ teaspoon of ginger, ground

Preparation:

Wash the cauliflower and trim off the outer leaves. Cut into small pieces and set aside.

Rinse the kale under cold running water and slightly drain. Torn with hands and set aside.

Wash the broccoli thoroughly and chop into small pieces. Set aside.

Wash the apple and cut lengthwise in half. remove the core and cut into bite-sized pieces. Set aside.

Now, combine cauliflower, kale, broccoli, cauliflower, apple and kale in a juicer and process until well juiced.

Transfer to a serving glass and stir in the ground ginger.

Enjoy!

Nutritional information per serving: Kcal: 131, Protein: 8.1g, Carbs: 36.8g, Fats: 1.5g

27.   Broccoli Grapes Juice

Ingredients:

1 cup of fresh broccoli, chopped

1 cup of green grapes

1 cup of cucumber, sliced

1 cup of mustard greens, torn

1 small ginger knob, peeled

2 oz of water

Preparation:

Wash the broccoli and cut into bite-sized pieces. Set aside.

Wash the grapes and set aside.

Wash the cucumber and cut into thin slices. Fill the measuring cup and reserve the rest for later.

Rinse the mustard greens thoroughly under cold running water. Torn with hands and set aside.

Peel the ginger knob and set aside.

Now, combine broccoli, grapes, cucumber, mustard greens and ginger in a juicer and process until juiced.

Transfer to a serving glass and stir in the water.

Add some ice and serve immediately.

Enjoy!

Nutritional information per serving: Kcal: 100, Protein: 5.2g, Carbs: 27.4g, Fats: 1g

28. Grape Watermelon Juice

Ingredients:

1 cup of green grapes

1 cup of watermelon, cubed

1 whole kiwi, peeled

1 medium-sized pear, chopped

¼ tsp of ceylon cinnamon, ground

Preparation:

Wash the grapes and set aside.

Cut the watermelon lengthwise. Cut one large wedge and peel it. Cut into chunks and fill the measuring cup. Remove the seeds and set aside. Reserve the rest of the melon for some other juices.

Peel the kiwi and cut lengthwise in half. Set aside.

Wash the pear and remove the core. Cut into bite-sized pieces and set aside.

Now, combine watermelon, grapes, kiwi, and pear in a juicer and process until well juiced.

Transfer to a serving glass and stir in the ceylon cinnamon

Enjoy!

Nutritional information per serving: Kcal: 216, Protein: 3g, Carbs: 64.5g, Fats: 1.2g

29. Cabbage Kale Kiwi Juice

Ingredients:

1 cup of cabbage, shredded

1 cup of fresh kale, torn

2 cups of fresh spinach, torn

1 cup of fresh parsley, torn

1 cup of cucumber, sliced

1 whole kiwi, peeled

1 cup of avocado, chunked

¼ tsp of turmeric, ground

Preparation:

Wash the cabbage thoroughly and shred the cabbage. Fill the measuring cup and reserve the rest for later.

Combine kale, spinach and parsley in a large colander. Rinse all under cold running water and slightly drain. Torn with hands and set aside.

Wash the cucumber and cut into thin slices. Set aside.

Peel the kiwi and cut lengthwise in half. Set aside

Peel the avocado and cut in half. Remove the pit and cut into small chunks. Fill the measuring cup and reserve the rest for later.

Now, combine cabbage, kale, spinach, parsley, cucumber, kiwi and avocado in a juicer and process until juiced.

Transfer to a serving glass and stir in the turmeric.

Refrigerate for 10 minutes and serve.

Enjoy!

Nutritional information per serving: Kcal: 290, Protein: 10.7g, Carbs: 40.3g, Fats: 23.1g

30.   Orange Beet Juice

Ingredients:

1 small blood orange, wedged

1 cup of beets, trimmed and sliced

1 cup of avocado, cubed

½ cup of green grapes

Preparation:

Peel the orange and divide into wedges. Cut each wedge in half and set aside.

Wash the beets thoroughly and trim off the green parts, Cut into thin slices and fill the measuring cup. Reserve the rest in the refrigerator. .

Peel the avocado and cut lengthwise in half. Cut into small cubes and fill the measuring cup. Reserve the rest for later.

Wash the grapes and fill the measuring cup. Set aside.

Now, combine orange, beets, avocado, and grapes in a juicer. Add few ice cubes and process until juiced.

Garnish with some fresh mint, if you like

Transfer to a serving glass and serve immediately.

Enjoy!

Nutrition information per serving: Kcal: 350, Protein: 7.3g, Carbs: 56.1g, Fats: 22.6g

31.   Grapes Cherry Juice

Ingredients:

1 cup of black grapes

1 cup of cherries, pitted

1 cup of blueberries

1 small blood orange, wedged

¼ tsp of cinnamon, ground

Preparation:

Wash the cherries and cut each in half. Remove the pits and set aside.

Combine blueberries and grapes in a colander and wash under cold running water. Slightly drain and set aside.

Peel the orange and divide into wedges. Cut each wedge in half and set aside.

Now, combine grapes, blueberries, cherries and orange in a juicer and process until juiced.

Transfer to a serving glass and stir in the cinnamon.

Add some ice and serve immediately.

Enjoy!

Nutritional information per serving: Kcal: 249, Protein: 4.2g, Carbs: 73.2g, Fats: 1.2g

32.   Avocado Broccoli Juice

Ingredients:

1 cup of avocado, cubed

1 cup of broccoli, chopped

1 medium-sized orange, peeled

1 cup of fresh kale, torn

2 large kiwis, peeled

Preparation:

Peel the avocado cut lengthwise in half. Remove the pit and cut into small cubes. Fill the measuring cup and reserve the rest for later. Set aside.

Wash the broccoli and cut into small pieces. Set aside.

Peel the orange and divide into wedges. Set aside.

Rinse the kale under cold running water and slightly drain. Torn with hands and set aside.

Peel the kiwis and cut lengthwise in half. Set aside.

Now, combine avocado, broccoli, orange,kale and kiwis under seeds in a juicer and process until juiced.

Transfer to a serving glass and add some ice before serving.

Garnish with some fresh mint, if you like. However, it's optional.

Enjoy!

Nutrition information per serving: Kcal: 357, Protein: 11.1g, Carbs: 59.9g, Fats: 23.2g

33. Spinach Kiwi Juice

Ingredients:

1 cup of fresh spinach, torn

¼ cup of fresh mint leaves

2 whole kiwis, peeled

1 small apple, cored

1 small peach, pitted

Preparation:

Rinse the spinach under cold running water and slightly drain. Torn with hands and set aside.

Combine spinach and mint in a large colander. Wash thoroughly under cold running water. Slightly drain and torn with hands. Set aside.

Peel the kiwis and cut lengthwise in half. Set aside.

Wash the apple and cut in half. Remove the core and cut into bite-sized pieces. Set aside.

Wash the peach and cut in half. Remove the pit and cut into bite-sized pieces. Set aside.

Now, combine spinach, kiwis, apple and peach in a juicer

and process until juiced. Transfer to a serving glass and add some ice.

Serve immediately.

Enjoy!

Nutrition information per serving: Kcal: 199, Protein: 5.3g, Carbs: 58.9g, Fats: 1.7g

34.   Orange Blackberry Juice

Ingredients:

1 medium-sized orange, peeled

1 cup of blackberries

1 cup of watermelon, cubed

1 tbsp of liquid honey

¼ tsp of cinnamon, ground

Preparation:

Peel the orange and divide into wedges. Cut each wedge in half and set aside.

Wash the blackberries thoroughly under cold water and slightly drain. Set aside.

Cut the watermelon in half. Cut one large wedge and wrap the rest in a plastic foil and refrigerate. Peel the slice and cut into small cubes. Remove the pits and fill the measuring cup. Set aside.

Wash the blackberries thoroughly under cold water and slightly drain. Set aside.

Now, combine watermelon, blackberries, and orange in a

juicer and process until juiced. Transfer to a serving glass and stir in the honey and cinnamon.

Refrigerate for 10 minutes before serving.

Enjoy!

Nutrition information per serving: Kcal: 186, Protein: 4.2g, Carbs: 40.7g, Fats: 1.1g

35.   Apples Grapes Green Juice

Ingredients:

2 medium sized Granny Smith apples, cored

1 cup of cucumber, sliced

17 green grapes

2 cup of fresh spinach, torn

Preparation:

Wash the apple and cut in half. Remove the core and cut into bite-sized pieces. Set aside.

Wash the cucumber and cut into thin slices. Fill the measuring cup and reserve the rest for later.

Wash the grapes and fill the measuring cup. Set aside.

Wash the spinach thoroughly and slightly drain. Torn with hands and set aside.

Now, combine apple, cucumber, grapes and spinach in a juicer and process until juiced.

Transfer to a serving glass . Garnish with some fresh mint, if you like. However, it's optional.

Enjoy!

Nutrition information per serving: Kcal: 127, Protein: 3.13g, Carbs: 33.77g, Fats: 0.79g

36.   Strawberry Mango Juice

Ingredients:

½ cup of strawberries, cut into bite-sized pieces

1 cup of mango, chunked

1 small apple, cored

2 whole cherries, pitted

1 tsp of dried mint, ground

Preparation:

Wash the strawberries and remove the core. Cut into bite-sized pieces and set aside.

Peel the mango and cut into bite-sized pieces. Set aside.

Wash the apple and cut in half. Remove the core and cut into small pieces. Set aside.

Wash the cherries and cut each in half. Remove the pits and set aside.

Place the mint in a small bowl and add two tablespoons of hot water. Let it soak for 5 minutes.

Now, combine mango, strawberries, apple, cherries and mint mixture in a juicer and process until juiced. Transfer to a serving glass and refrigerate for 15 minutes before serving.

Enjoy!

Nutritional information per serving: Kcal: 185, Protein: 2.8g, Carbs: 53.8g, Fats: 1.1g

37.   Kale Broccoli Juice

Ingredients:

2 cups of kale, roughly chopped

2 cups of broccoli, chopped

2 medium-sized asparagus spears, trimmed

1 cup of fresh mint, torn

1 whole lemon, peeled

1 small ginger knob, peeled

Preparation:

Rinse the kale under cold running water. Slightly drain and torn with hands. Set aside.

Trim off the outer leaves of the broccoli. Wash it and cut into bite-sized pieces. Set aside.

Wash the asparagus and trim off the woody ends. Cut into small pieces and set aside.

Wash the mint and roughly chop it. You can soak it in water for 5 minutes before preparation, but it's optional. Set aside.

Peel the ginger knob and set aside.

Peel the lemon and cut lengthwise in half. Set aside.

Now, combine broccoli, kale, asparagus, ginger, mint, and lemon in a juicer. Process until juiced. Transfer to a serving glass and refrigerate for 15 minutes before serving.

Enjoy!

Nutritional information per serving: Kcal: 118, Protein: 13.3g, Carbs: 35.3g, Fats: 2.4g

38.   Apple Celery Juice

Ingredients:

1 large green apple, cored

1 large lemon, peeled

3 large celery stalks, chopped

1 large cucumber

2 oz of coconut water

Preparation:

Wash the apple and cut lengthwise in half. Remove the core and cut into small chunks. Set aside.

Peel the lemon and cut lengthwise in half. Set aside.

Wash the celery stalks and cut into small pieces. Set aside.

Peel the cucumber and cut into small chunks. Set aside.

Now, combine apple, lemon, celery, and cucumber in a juicer and process until well juiced. Transfer to serving glasses and stir in the coconut water.

Add few ice cubes and serve immediately.

Enjoy!

Nutritional information per serving: Kcal: 175, Protein: 5.1g, Carbs: 50.2g, Fats: 1.3g

39.   Kale Carrot Juice

Ingredients:

1 cup of fresh kale, chopped

1 large carrot, sliced

1 large celery, chopped

1 small Granny Smith's apple, cored

1 tbsp of liquid honey

Preparation:

Rinse the kale under cold running water using a colander. Slightly drain and torn with hands. Set aside.

Wash and peel the carrot. Cut into thin slices and set aside.

Wash the celery and cut into bite-sized pieces. Set aside.

Wash the apple and cut lengthwise in half. Remove the core and cut into bite-sized pieces. Set aside.

Now, combine kale,carrot, celery, and apple in a juicer and process until juiced. Transfer to a serving glass and stir in the honey.

Add some ice and serve immediately.

Enjoy!

Nutritional information per serving: Kcal: 179, Protein: 4.6g, Carbs: 34.3g, Fats: 1.1g

40. Fennel Spinach Juice

Ingredients:

1 cup of fennel, chopped

1 cup of collard greens, torn

3 large green apples, cored

1 cup of fresh spinach, torn

Preparation:

Wash the fennel bulb and trim off the wilted outer layers. Cut into small chunks and fill the measuring cup. Reserve the rest in the refrigerator.

In a large colander, combine collard greens and spinach. Rinse thoroughly under cold running water and drain. Torn with hands and set aside.

Wash the apples and cut in half. Remove the core and cut into bite-sized pieces. Set aside.

Now, combine fennel, collard greens, spinach and apple in a juicer. Process until well juiced.

Transfer to a serving glass and refrigerate for 15 minutes before serving.

Enjoy!

Nutritional information per serving: Kcal: 220, Protein: 5g, Carbs: 66.3g, Fats: 1.3g

41.   Cucumber Broccoli Juice

Ingredients:

1 cup of cucumber, sliced

2 cups of broccoli, chopped

1 cup of Brussels sprouts

1 teaspoon of olive oil

Preparation:

Wash the cucumber and cut into thin slices. Fill the measuring cup and reserve the rest for later. Set aside.

Wash the broccoli and trim off the outer layers. Cut into small pieces and set aside.

Wash the Brussels sprouts and trim off the outer wilted leaves. Cut in half and set aside.

Now, combine Cucumber, Broccoli and Brussels sprouts in a juicer and process until well juiced and add one teaspoon of olive oil before serving.

Serve immediately.

Enjoy!

Nutrition information per serving: Kcal: 74, Protein: 8.4g, Carbs: 21.8g, Fats: 1g

42. Cauliflower Broccoli Juice

Ingredients:

1 cup of cauliflower, chopped

1 cup of fresh basil, torn

2 cups of broccoli, chopped

1 medium-sized red apple, cored

1 large lemon, peeled

Preparation:

Trim off the outer leaves of a cauliflower. Wash it and fill and cut into small pieces. Fill the measuring cup and reserve the rest in the refrigerator.

Wash the broccoli and chop into small pieces. Set aside.

Wash the apple and cut lengthwise in half. Remove the core and cut into bite-sized pieces. Set aside.

Peel the lemon and cut lengthwise in half. Set aside.

Now, combine cauliflower, basil, broccoli, apple and lemon in a juicer. Process until well juiced and transfer to a serving glass.

Add few ice cubes and serve immediately.

Enjoy!

Nutritional information per serving: Kcal: 156, Protein: 9g, Carbs: 46.4g, Fats: 1.5g

43.   Zucchini Basil Juice

Ingredients:

1 small zucchini, chopped

1 cup of mustard greens, chopped

2 cups of fresh basil, chopped

1 whole lime, peeled

1 whole cucumber, sliced

Preparation:

Peel the zucchini and cut into bite-sized pieces. Set aside.

Combine fresh basil and mustard greens in a large colander. Wash thoroughly under cold running water. Roughly chop it and soak in lukewarm water for 10 minutes.

Peel the lime and cut lengthwise in half. Set aside.

Wash the cucumber and cut into thin slices. Set aside.

Now, combine zucchini, basil, mustard greens, lime, and cucumber in a juicer and process until well juiced. Transfer to a serving glass and refrigerate for 10 minutes before serving.

Enjoy!

Nutritional information per serving: Kcal: 126, Protein: 7.5g, Carbs: 38.8g, Fats: 1.4g

44.   Cauliflower Avocado Juice

Ingredients:

5 cauliflower flowerets, chopped

1 cup of avocado, cubed

1 whole lime, peeled

1 whole leek, chopped

Preparation:

Wash the cauliflower flowerets thoroughly and chop into small pieces. Set aside.

Peel the avocado and cut in half. Remove the pit and cut into small cubes. Fill the measuring cup and reserve the rest in the refrigerator. Set aside.

Peel the lime and cut lengthwise in half. Set aside.

Wash the leek and cut into small pieces. Set aside.

Now, combine cauliflower, avocado, lime, and leek in a juicer and process until juiced. Transfer to a serving glass and refrigerate for 10 minutes before serving.

Enjoy!

Nutritional information per serving: Kcal: 268, Protein: 5.7g, Carbs: 32.4g, Fats: 22.5g

45.   Apple Kale Juice

Ingredients:

1 medium-sized red apple, cored

1 cup of cucumber, sliced

2 cups of fresh kale, chopped

1 cup of watercress, torn

1 cup of fresh parsley, torn

1 oz of water

Preparation:

Wash the cucumber and cut into thin slices. Fill the measuring cup and reserve the rest for later. Set aside.

Wash the apple and cut lengthwise in half. Remove the core and cut into bite-sized pieces. Set aside.

Wash the kale thoroughly under cold running water. Chop into small pieces and set aside.

Combine watercress and parsley in a colander. Rinse well under cold running water and torn with hands. Set aside.

Now, combine cucumber, apple, kale, watercress, and parsley in a juicer and process until juiced. Transfer to a serving glass and stir in the water. Add some ice before serving.

Enjoy!

Nutritional information per serving: Kcal: 150, Protein: 9.1g, Carbs: 40.8g, Fats: 2g

46.   Carrots Orange Juice

Ingredients:

2 medium-sized carrots, sliced

2 cups of broccoli, chopped

1 large orange, peeled

1 whole lemon, peeled

1 small ginger knob, peeled

Preparation:

Wash and peel the carrot. Cut into thin slices and set aside.

Trim off the outer leaves of the broccoli. Wash it and cut into bite-sized pieces. Set aside.

Peel the orange and divide into wedges. Cut each wedge in half and set aside.

Peel the lemon and cut lengthwise in half. Set aside.

Peel the ginger knob and set aside.

Now, combine carrots, broccoli, orange, lemon, and, ginger knob in a juicer. Process until juiced.

Transfer to a serving glass and refrigerate for 15 minutes before serving.

Nutritional information per serving: Kcal: 162, Protein: 8.7g, Carbs: 51.8g, Fats: 1.4g

47.   Kale Broccoli Juice

Ingredients:

1 cup of kale, roughly chopped

2 cups of broccoli, chopped

1 small green apple, cored

1 medium-sized asparagus spears, trimmed

1 whole lemon, peeled

1 cup of fresh parsley, torn

Preparation:

Rinse the kale under cold running water. Slightly drain and torn with hands. Set aside.

Trim off the outer leaves of the broccoli. Wash it and cut into bite-sized pieces. Set aside.

Wash the apple and cut in half. Remove the core and cut into bite-sized pieces. Set aside.

Wash the asparagus and trim off the woody ends. Cut into small pieces and set aside.

Peel the lemon and cut lengthwise in half. Set aside.

Add parsley in a colander. Rinse well under cold running water and torn with hands. Set aside.

Now, combine kale, broccoli, apple, asparagus, lemon and parsley in a juicer. Process until juiced.

Transfer to a serving glass and refrigerate for 15 minutes before serving.

Nutritional information per serving: Kcal: 154, Protein: 11.1g, Carbs: 45.3g, Fats: 2.1g

48.   Zucchini Parsnip Juice

Ingredients:

1 cup of cucumber, sliced

1 small zucchini, chopped

1 cup of parsnip, sliced

1 medium-sized carrot, sliced

¼ tsp of ginger, ground

Preparation:

Wash the cucumber and cut into slices. Fill the measuring cup and reserve the rest for later.

Peel the zucchini and cut into bite-sized pieces. Set aside.

Wash and slightly peel the parsnip. Cut into thin slices and fill the measuring cup. Reserve the rest for later. Set aside.

Wash and peel the carrot. Cut into thin slices and set aside.

Now, combine cucumber, zucchini, parsnip and carrot in a juicer and process until juiced.

Transfer to a serving glass and stir in the ginger. Refrigerate for 10 minutes before serving.

Enjoy!

Nutritional information per serving: Kcal: 161, Protein: 7g, Carbs: 48.1g, Fats 1.8g

49.   Carrot Apple Juice

Ingredients:

2 large carrots, sliced

2 small green apples, cored

1 small zucchini, chopped

1 large lime, peeled

¼ tsp of ginger, ground

Preparation:

Wash and peel the carrots. Cut into thin slices and set aside.

Wash the apple and cut in half. Remove the core and cut into bite-sized pieces. Set aside.

Peel the zucchini and cut into thin slices. Set aside.

Peel the lime and cut lengthwise in half. Set aside.

Now, combine carrots, apples, zucchini and lime in a juicer. Process until well juiced. Transfer to a serving glass and stir in the ginger.

Enjoy!

Nutritional information per serving: Kcal: 161, Protein: 7g, Carbs: 48.1g, Fats: 1.8g

50. Raspberries Basil Juice

Ingredients:

2 medium-sized carrots, sliced

2 cups of raspberries

1 cup of fresh basil, torn

1 whole lemon, peeled

1 small Granny Smith's apple, cored

Preparation:

Wash and peel the carrots. Cut into thin slices and set aside.

Using a colander, rinse the raspberries under cold running water. Slightly drain and set aside.

Wash the basil thoroughly and torn with hands. Set aside.

Peel the lemon and cut lengthwise in half. Set aside.

Wash the apple and cut in half. Remove the core and cut into bite-sized pieces. Set aside.

Now, combine carrots, raspberries, basil, lemon and apple in a juicer and process until juiced.

Transfer to a serving glass and add few ice cubes.

Serve immediately.

Enjoy!

Nutritional information per serving: Kcal: 223, Protein: 7.3g, Carbs: 79.5g, Fats: 2.8g

51. Raspberry Carrot Juice

Ingredients:

1 cup of raspberries

1 cup of blackberries

1 cup of blueberries

2 large carrots, peeled and chopped

1 large orange, wedged

1 tsp of fresh rosemary, finely chopped

Preparation:

Using a colander, wash the raspberries in under cold running water. Slightly drain and set aside.

Combine blackberries and blueberries in a colander. Rinse under cold running water and drain. Set aside.

Wash the carrots and peel them. Cut into small chunks and set aside.

Peel the orange and divide into wedges. Set aside.

Now, combine raspberries, blueberries, blackberries, carrots, orange and rosemary in a juicer and process until well juiced. Transfer to a serving glass.

Refrigerate for 10 minutes before serving.

Nutritional information per serving: Kcal: 246, Protein: 7.6g, Carbs: 85.4g, Fats: 2.5g

52.   Collard greens Carrot Juice

Ingredients:

2 cup of cucumber, sliced

2 cups of collard greens, torn

1 cup of fresh parsley, chopped

3 medium-sized carrots, sliced

1 tsp of fresh rosemary, finely chopped

Preparation:

Wash the cucumber and cut into thin slices. Fill the measuring cup and reserve the rest for later. Set aside.

Wash the collard greens thoroughly under cold running water. Place them in a bowl and add 2 cups of boiling water. Let it soak for 10 minutes. Slightly drain and set aside.

Rinse the parsley under cold running water and chop into small pieces.

Wash and peel the carrot. Cut into thin slices and set aside.

Now, combine cucumber, collard greens, parsley, carrots, and rosemary in a juicer and process until juiced.

Transfer to a serving glass and refrigerate for 10 minutes before serving.

Nutritional information per serving: Kcal: 94, Protein: 6.3g, Carbs: 29g, Fats: 1.4g

53. Avocado Collard Greens Juice

Ingredients

1 cup of avocado, cubed

2 cups of collard greens, torn

1 small Granny Smith's apple, cored

1 cup of watercress, torn

1 tsp of fresh rosemary, finely chopped

Preparation:

Peel the avocado and cut in half. Remove the pit and cut into small cubes. Fill the measuring cup and reserve the rest in the refrigerator. Set aside.

Wash the collard greens thoroughly under cold running water. Place them in a bowl and add 2 cups of boiling water. Let it soak for 10 minutes. Slightly drain and set aside.

Wash the apple and cut in half. Remove the core and cut into bite-sized pieces. Set aside.

Wash the watercress and torn with hands. Set aside.

Now, combine avocado, collard greens, apples, watercress

and rosemary in a juicer.

Process until well juiced and transfer to a serving glass. Refrigerate for 10 minutes before serving.

Nutritional information per serving: Kcal: 389, Protein: 8.1g, Carbs: 43.5g, Fats: 34.4g

54.   Mixed Berry Juice

Ingredients:

1 cup of cranberries

1 cup of blackberries

1 cup of blueberries

1 large lime, peeled

1 large cucumber, chopped

1 cup of parsnip, sliced

Preparation:

Combine cranberries, blackberries and blueberries in a colander. Rinse under cold running water and drain. Set aside.

Peel the lime and cut lengthwise in half. Set aside.

Wash the cucumber and cut into small chunks. Set aside.

Wash and slightly peel the parsnip. Cut into thin slices and fill the measuring cup. Reserve the rest for later. Set aside.

Now, combine cranberries, blackberries, blueberries, cucumber, lime and parsnip in a juicer and process until juiced. Transfer to serving glasses and stir in the water.

Add some ice or refrigerate for 15 minutes before serving.

Nutritional information per serving: Kcal: 243, Protein: 7g, Carbs: 82.3g, Fats: 2g

55.   Apple Cranberry Juice

Ingredients:

1 small Granny Smith's apple, chopped

1 cup of cranberries

1 cup of watercress, torn

½ cup of fresh spinach, torn

1 small ginger knob, peeled

Preparation:

Wash the apple and remove the core. Cut into bite-sized pieces and set aside.

Place the cranberries in a colander and rinse thoroughly. Slightly drain and set aside.

Wash watercress and spinach thoroughly under cold running water. Drain and torn with hands. Set aside.

Peel the ginger and set aside.

Now, combine apple, cranberries, watercress, spinach, and ginger in a juicer and process until well juiced. Transfer to a serving glass and stir in some water if you like. However, it is optional.

Refrigerate for 15 minutes before serving.

Enjoy!

Nutritional information per serving: Kcal: 249, Protein: 3.8g, Carbs: 86.1g, Fats: 0.9g

56.   Fennel Collard Green Juice

Ingredients:

1 cup of fennel, chopped

1 cup of collard greens, torn

1 large green apple, cored

A handful of spinach

1 teaspoon of olive oil

Preparation:

Wash the fennel bulb and trim off the wilted outer layers. Cut into small chunks and fill the measuring cup. Reserve the rest in the refrigerator.

In a large colander, combine collard greens and spinach. Rinse thoroughly under cold running water and drain. Torn with hands and set aside.

Wash the apple and cut in half. Remove the core and cut into bite-sized pieces. Set aside.

Now, combine fennel, collard greens, spinach, and apple in a juicer. Process until well juiced.

Transfer to a serving glass and add one teaspoon of olive

oil and refrigerate for 15 minutes before serving.

Enjoy!

Nutritional information per serving: Kcal: 122, Protein: 3.9g, Carbs: 37.4g, Fats: 0.9g

57.   Avocado Kale Juice

Ingredients:

1 cup of fresh spinach, torn

1 cup of fresh kale, torn

1 cup of fresh parsley, torn

1 cup of cucumber, sliced

1 cup of avocado, chunked

¼ tsp of turmeric, ground

Preparation:

Combine spinach, kale, and parsley in a large colander. Rinse all under cold running water and slightly drain. Torn with hands and set aside.

Wash the cucumber and cut into thin slices. Set aside.

Peel the avocado and cut in half. Remove the pit and cut into small chunks. Fill the measuring cup and reserve the rest for later.

Now, combine spinach, kale, parsley, cucumber and avocado in a juicer and process until juiced. Transfer to a serving glass and stir in the turmeric.

Refrigerate for 10 minutes and serve.

Enjoy!

Nutritional information per serving: Kcal: 285, Protein: 17.3g, Carbs: 34.8g, Fats: 24.4g

ADDITIONAL TITLES FROM THIS AUTHOR

70 Effective Meal Recipes to Prevent and Solve Being Overweight: Burn Fat Fast by Using Proper Dieting and Smart Nutrition

By

Joe Correa CSN

48 Acne Solving Meal Recipes: The Fast and Natural Path to Fixing Your Acne Problems in Less Than 10 Days!

By

Joe Correa CSN

41 Alzheimer's Preventing Meal Recipes: Reduce or Eliminate Your Alzheimer's Condition in 30 Days or Less!

By

Joe Correa CSN

70 Effective Breast Cancer Meal Recipes: Prevent and Fight Breast Cancer with Smart Nutrition and Powerful Foods

By

Joe Correa CSN

www.ingramcontent.com/pod-product-compliance
Lightning Source LLC
Chambersburg PA
CBHW030244030426
42336CB00009B/252